I0439250

35 Best Ways to Save Money When You Have Cancer

Julie L. Kaye

The Health Correspondent
c/o Julie L. Kaye
P.O. Box 235745
Encinitas, CA 92023

©The Health Correspondent by Julie L. Kaye 2013

ISBN-13 9781494867959

Book cover designed by Angie Zambrano. 1st Edition

To my beautiful, wonderful and wise daughter Eleanor Xin Hua Lian who learned at a very young age that people can be just like Legos - while they may fall apart, they can also be rebuilt.

To my father who showed me a childhood filled with beauty, art and travel and whom I love very dearly.

To my mother Diane whose own cancer forced me to become an adult over night and start shifting my focus from myself to others.

To my Aunt Judy and Uncle Marty who loved me unconditionally and I will be forever grateful.

TABLE OF CONTENTS

Introduction

How To Get The Medical Care You Need

Medicaid And Cancer

How to Get Your Co-Pays, Premiums and Deductibles Paid by Medicaid

How To Save On Your Hospital Bills

How To Have Your Medical Bills Checked For Errors For Free

Where To Find The Most Comprehensive Information On Medication Assistance

How To Find Discounts On MRI's And CAT Scans

Programs To Mediate Medical Bills

The Affordable Care Act And Your Rights As Someone With Cancer

How To Get A Free Estimate On Your Cost In The Upcoming Marketplace

Where To Find Free Assistance Creating A Debt Management Program

How To Lower Many Of Your Monthly Expenses

How To Reduce The Fat From Your Grocery Bills

Where To Find Free And Low Cost Delivered Meals

How To Find Free Short, Medium, And Long Distance Transportation

How To Find Free And Low Cost Complementary Medicine

Where To Find Free And Lower Cost Genetic Testing

How To Get Your Home Cleaned For Free (For Women Only)

How To Go On A Free Cruise If You Have Cancer Or Are Recovering

How To Get A Free Spa Certificate If You Are A Woman Who Has Cancer

Where To Order The Most Beautiful Silk Head Wraps For Free

How To Get Free Gift Cards When You Have Cancer

Introduction

The information in this booklet is what I needed when I had cancer. Most of it wasn't available at the time, and has only just become so. When I was diagnosed with breast cancer in November of 2008, I was a single mother of a hyper active four year little girl who needed to be on one of those puppy leashes.

We had just moved back to San Diego after spending a year in New York, so I could be near my father after my divorce and child custody battle. I had temporarily put myself on a low cost health insurance plan that covered nine doctor's visits per year, but not major medical. What was I thinking? I thought I could get by for one year on a cheaper plan.

We were staying with a friend while I was looking for work. I was told I had breast cancer by my physician , before I found a job. My friend was more upset than I was about my cancer diagnosis. She told people we had cancer.

On a personal note, my friend is a great person, but couldn't deal with cancer. She did help with my daughter. Just think about it, you and your child are invited to go stay at a friend's house, and you're told that you have cancer, and you have no home to go back to.

We moved several times that year and I negotiated every bill I had. Put it this way, I had no time to think about the cancer; I was too busy trying to get by and take care of my daughter.

That year was so tough that I considered the five surgeries I had and chemotherapy to be like spa treatments. I got to relax, well kind of. Even while I was going through treatments, I was making mental notes of my experiences. I kept asking myself, "Could I be the only one going through this financial black hole during cancer? "

This booklet is written for people who have cancer and need quick financial relief. Many cancer websites and non-profit organizations make grant applications available for "limited" financial assistance. You will need to be patient because they have a long list of people waiting and the check will probably be $100-$200 for a gas card or bus fare. While this amount will undoubtedly be useful, I doubt it will be enough to reduce your financial stress over the long term.

I applied to numerous organizations for help considering that no one was going to hire me while I was going through cancer treatment. It turns out that many organizations were listed as having funds but they ran out, closed down, I didn't fit their criteria, or I just never heard from them. The one organization that came through was Susan J. Komen

Foundation. They directed me to Breast Cancer Solutions of San Diego which is currently a 2012-2013 Grantee.

There is unquestionably more help for breast cancer patients than any other type of cancer. Nevertheless, people with all cancers need to know where to turn for financial assistance without making that search a full time job.

My uncle once said to me "Julie if you live long enough you will see it all." From The Affordable Care Act, to affordable programs to subsidize the cost of medicine, access of vital information for patients, genetic testing becoming accessible to the masses and so many new laws to protect millions of Americans, help is available if you know where to look.

How To Get The Medical Care You Need

When you are first diagnosed with cancer, one of the first alarms that go off in your mind is, can I pay for this help or will I be wiped out? Hopefully this advice will alleviate those fears. Go to the Patient's Financial Services Department of your hospital and ask the manager of patient accounts what options you have. This is exactly what I did and ended up telling all of San Diego on Channel 8 News.

Just asking people who deal with this every day should open opportunities you didn't think existed. If you are uninsured or underinsured but not considered low income, you can still receive substantial discounts, especially if you ask before surgeries, chemo, radiation, etc...

Don't forget to ask what other billers you should contact who will be involved in your care and therefore billing you. Some hospitals and medical providers will negotiate a 35% to 40% discount for uninsured patients, but you need to ask for it, says Candice Butcher, the CEO of Medical Billing Advocates of America. Once you have negotiated the price for your procedure or procedures please do not leave without the agreement in writing signed and dated. Make a copy and leave it somewhere safe!

If you are told that you don't qualify for government assistance, you may still qualify for charity care programs offered by hospitals and doctors offices. Speak with a financial counselor or manager of patient accounts to see if you meet their qualifications.

The information below is also essential information:

Hill-Burton Hospital Program
www.hrsa.gov
800-638-0742

http://www.hrsa.gov/gethealthcare/affordable/hillburton/hillburton.pdf

Hospitals that receive construction funds from the federal government must provide some services to cancer patients who can't afford to pay for their care. Approximately 165 hospitals and medical facilities take part in this program. Once they complete their obligation to the government the facility is removed from the list, so the list is constantly being updated. Please look at the .pdf listed above to find a participating hospital in your area.

Some hospitals won't recognize The Hill Burton Program, just ask them what charity programs are available and if they will help you apply. Also ask them how fast decisions are made for people already diagnosed with cancer.

How To Contact Medicare's State Health Assistance Programs To Get The Help You Need

There are Medicare information centers ready to help you understand your plan and help you get what you need. I called the state Medicare office in Florida since that state has a high concentration of seniors. I expected to get a recording or be put on hold, but someone picked up the phone right away and couldn't have been more helpful. The .pdf below lists the contact information by the state. The state help line will direct you to your local office.

http://www.hapnetwork.org/assets/pdfs/state-ship-contact-information.pdf

Medicaid And Cancer

Medicaid is subject to your state cancer coverage laws and the laws governing clinical trials. What this means is that if your state covers "off-label" use of cancer drugs and/or clinical trials, you are covered as a Medicaid cancer patient. "Off Label" is a term referring to a drug being used for something other than what it was originally intended to be used for.

As it turns out, 50 to 75% of cancer drugs are used "off label," and this practice is widely accepted among oncologists, government agencies and insurance carriers. You have every right to ask your oncologist about the chemotherapy he/she is planning on using. For instance how effective is it for your type of cancer? Are there studies to support the findings that you could read? Here is an interesting article from Consumer Reports:

http://www.consumerreports.org/health/resources/pdf/best-buy-drugs/money-saving-guides/english/Off-Label-FINAL.pdf

The bottom of the article discusses cancer drugs & "off label" uses.

If you are trying to get Medicaid Coverage, your hospital and/or local Medicaid office should do everything in their power to help you. Just in case you are still having problems getting covered, you may well be able to sign up for the expanded Medicaid coverage under the Affordable Care Act starting October 1, 2013. The effective starting date will be Jan. 1, 2014. Meanwhile, there are many available options for help over the next several pages!

How to Get Your Co-Pays, Premiums and Deductibles Paid by Medicaid

HIPP aka Health Insurance Premium Payment Program

disabilityrightslegalcenter.org

866-843-2572

HIPP is a Medicaid Program that pays co-pays, premiums, and deductible for employees of companies who have high medical costs due to a health condition. The employee must have group insurance or access to group health insurance through their employer at the time of application, have a medical condition which is covered by their health insurance plan and have at least one member of your family on Medicaid. It is available in the following states;

Iowa, Texas, Pennsylvania, California, Alabama, Colorado, Idaho, Georgia, Kentucky, Illinois, Louisiana, Minnesota, Missouri, Nebraska, Rhode Island, South Carolina, Virginia, New Hampshire, West Virginia, Oregon, Wisconsin.

Coverage For All

www.coverageforall.org

Coverage For All, sponsored by The Foundation for Health Coverage Education is a fantastic resource for all Americans. By answering a few simple questions you can immediately find out exactly which government sponsored or private program is best suited for you and how to apply.

How To Save On Your Hospital Bills

When a hospital bill isn't paid or paid in full, the bill can get turned over to a collection agency. The collection agencies typically receives up to 25% of what has been reclaimed, according to Dr. Mark Friedman, the founder of billing consultant Premium HealthCare Services. That's your first insight into the initial amount of lee-way in the bill.

The site "www.healthcarebluebook.com" is a gold mine for patients. It shows you as the healthcare consumer how to easily check Health Care prices by ZIP code. Did you ever think about shopping for the best "fee for service" on top of quality? This is especially important when you are having multiple procedures and treatments over an extended period of time.

According to The Healthcare Blue Book, providers frequently charge uninsured cash paying customers 2-5 times more than what they accept from an insurance company for the same service. Even if you have insurance but are paying for part of your treatment (deductible or co-insurance), you could be charged a wide range of network prices for the same service. A recent Thompson Healthcare study reported that insurers frequently pay between $500 and $3,000 for the same MRI. Choosing the best provider can save you $2,500 or more.

How To Have Your Medical Bills Checked For Errors For Free

Medical billing mistakes can be costly if they go undetected. According to medical experts, 40% to 80% of medical bills contain errors, and Kaiser Health News estimates that nearly $68 billion in health care spending is lost to fraud and billing mistakes every year.

To help consumers combat errors and keep more money in their pockets medical website Simplee.com launched a new service that identifies mistakes on medical bills. There's enough external evidence that a high percentage of medical bills contain errors in them,says Tomer Shoval, co-founder and chief executive of simplee.com. In the past billing mistakes weren't a big deal to consumers because insurance typically covered all their medical costs which is not the case today.

Where To Find The Most Comprehensive Information On Medication Assistance

The Association of Community Cancer Center's 2013 Digital Edition of The Patient Assistance and Reimbursement Guide.

This digital edition brings together information on PAP's (Patient Assistance Programs) and Reimbursement Resources.

ACCC's highly praised and valuable resource:

http://www.accc-cancer.org/publications/PatientAssistanceGuide.asp

This guide features a list of pharmaceutical and non-pharmaceutical patient assistance programs. It provides a quick reference guide with links directly to the drug manufacturers by drug name and directions on how to apply to patient assistance programs and links to enrollment forms.

How To Find Discounts On MRI's And CAT Scans

Program for MRI & CAT Scan Discounts offered by **NeedyMeds**

http://www.needymeds.org/indices/imaging_discount_servic e_landing_pa

800-503-6897

Programs To Mediate Medical Bills

http://www.needymeds.org/indices/medical_mediation.htm

http://www.healthproponent.com

866-939-3435

Health Proponent offers a membership of $24.95 for the year and $99 per case.

The Affordable Care Act And Your Rights As Someone With Cancer

This book is being written and published before the official information and rates are determined for the new policies being offered through The Affordable Care Act.; but I will include what I understand so far.

No matter what state you live in, you'll be able to use the Marketplace to apply for coverage, compare your options, and enroll. Most people will be eligible for health coverage through the Health Insurance Marketplace.

To be eligible for health coverage through the Marketplace, you:

must live in the United States
must be a U.S. citizen or national (or be lawfully present) can't be currently incarcerated.

There is an easy to use scroll down menu listing states to learn about the Marketplace that will serve you.

Starting in 2014, health insurance plans can't refuse to cover you or charge you more just because you have a pre-existing health condition.

To clarify, an insurance company can't turn you down or charge you more because you have cancer. Once you have insurance, it can't refuse to cover your cancer treatments. Coverage for your type of cancer begins immediately. This is true even if you have been turned down or refused coverage because of cancer previously.

One exception: Grandfathered individual health insurance plans

If you have a pre-existing condition and are covered under Medicare, Medicaid or the Children's Health Insurance Program (CHIP) they also can't refuse to cover you or charge you more. Also, you will not need to re-enroll in the Marketplace, since you are already enrolled in one of these programs

Questions? Call 1-800-318-2596, 24 hours a day, 7 days a week. (TTY: 1-855-889-4325) or go to www.healthcare.gov

You can apply for insurance in The Health Insurance Marketplace when open enrollment starts on October 1, 2013. Coverage starts as soon as January 1, 2014. Open enrollment ends on March 31, 2014. Outside of open enrollment, you can't enroll in Marketplace coverage unless you have a qualifying life event.

How To Get A Free Estimate On Your Cost In The Upcoming Marketplace

The Kaiser Family Foundation has developed a health insurance cost and savings calculator in the link below. It is only an estimate. Your final premiums and costs may differ from the estimates, perhaps significantly, depending on where you live and the coverage you select. You'll learn your final costs for specific plans when you apply in the Health Insurance Marketplace as soon as October 1, 2013.

The calculator was created by the Kaiser Family Foundation, a non-profit research organization, for use by the general public. The Kaiser Family Foundation is solely responsible for the tool. The Kaiser Family Foundation has no connection with Kaiser Permanente or any health care provider. Before you use the Kaiser Family Foundation calculator, there are a few important things to know:

The calculator provides a rough estimate of costs for insurance, based on national averages and factors that may not apply to you. It will give you an idea of what someone with circumstances like yours could pay for Marketplace insurance in 2014.

The calculator accounts for some factors that may determine plan costs in the Marketplace: age, family size, and tobacco use. Individual plans will weigh these factors differently to determine final prices.

The estimate doesn't account for differences based on where you live, which will significantly affect Marketplace prices and offerings. The prices are based on a plan in the Silver category. Plans in different categories will likely have higher or lower premiums.

You won't be able to get your exact costs for a specific plan until you fill out a Marketplace application after October 1, 2013. Then you'll see all of the plans available to you, compare features and prices side-by-side, choose a plan, and enroll. You should expect that your final cost will be different from the rough estimate provided here.

http://kff.org/interactive/subsidy-calculator/

The Centers for Medicare & Medicaid Services did not participate in the creation of this calculator. The Centers for Medicare & Medicaid Services does not warrant or guarantee the accuracy of estimates provided by the calculator.

Where To Find Free Assistance Creating A Debt Management Program

Money Management International
www.moneymanagement.org
tel:866.889.9347

MMI is a valuable service for people who need help reducing their expenses and managing the money they have. One example of what they can do for you is by creating a Debt Management Plan to help you repay your debt. A Debt Management Plan is recommended for those individuals who need more than advice and could benefit from a structured repayment plan.

Through a Debt Management Plan, you are able to make one convenient monthly deposit to MMI which is then disbursed to each of your creditors. A Debt Management Plan may help:

Reduce interest rates
Waive late fees
Lower monthly payments Eliminate collection calls

Counselors are available 24 hours a day, 7 days a week by telephone and Internet. In-person credit counseling is also available by appointment in the local markets listed on their website. To get started, fill out the online counseling form or call to speak with a certified credit counselor about the options available to you.

How To Lower Many Of Your Monthly Expenses

There are lots of ways to quickly lower your monthly expenses:

Telecommunications Bills (AT&T, Cox, Time Warner, Comcast) make an enormous amount of money telling people they need these bloated packages of cable, Internet and phone and additional add-ons. My suggestion is to think about what you really use versus what you don't. Do you really use all 500 channels plus HBO and Showtime?

Are you really using your home phone and do you need the fastest high speed internet? Ask your customer service representative to tell you what lower priced packages they are offering at the moment and also how much would it be if you didn't have a package and you got the lower priced levels for Internet, cable, etc. For instance you could go to a slower high speed Internet. I can almost guarantee that most of you won't know the difference. You can probably lower your bill while you're on the phone speaking to the representative.

I have reduced many telecommunications bills for people and it's very possible to save $40-$75 per month. While this might not sound earth shattering to you, it adds up. This is $480-$900 per year in savings.

Cell Phones & Cell Phone Contracts (AT&T, Verizon, Sprint)

Cell Phone contracts are thought of as Iron Clad and if you want or need to get out the contract before the two years is up, you will need to pay at least $150. This is not accurate for people who have cancer though. I called up the three giants in this field and this is what I was told:

For **Verizon** call customer service at **1-800-922-0204**. Tell them that you have cancer, and ask to cancel your contract immediately. They will not ask you for any details.

For **AT&T** call **1-800-288-0500**. Ask for Customer Relations, and tell them that you have an "economic health hardship" due to your cancer and to please cancel your contract. They will not ask any details or require anything in writing.

Sprint's # is **888-211-4727**. Their fax # is **866-766-2791**. Sprint will not only cancel your contract if you have cancer; they will pay your current balance according to Angelica the account manager I spoke to in account services. They ask that you call account services first, and have your doctor's office fax a letter or proof of your diagnosis.

Lower cost cellular prepaid programs are easy to find now. Some examples are:

Verizon Prepaid Programs which range from $35 per month to $90 per month. Contact or visit your local Verizon store to learn more.

Straight Talk

www.straighttalk.com **855-222-2355**

Straighttalk offers unlimited phone, texting and Internet. Their cell phone programs range from $30 per month using straighttalk phones for 1000 minutes, 1000 texts and free 411, $45 per month for unlimited talk, text, Internet, 411 or $60 a month for unlimited international phone, text, Internet, 411 using your own GSM or CDMA phone. Contact your provider to determine what type of phone you have.

* Their phones require buying a Straight Talk SIM card (ask customer service which SIM card you need for your phone) and an unlocked phone. The sim card will be mailed to you within a week of ordering. If your phone isn't unlocked, you can easily find someone on Craigslist do it for $10-$15.

I have been using Straight Talk for about a year. This service is fantastic and so are their rates. I recommend paying monthly but not using their automatic payment deduction. Their system has charged me for a few months at a time.

PagePlus Cellular

www.pagepluscellular.com **800-550-2436**

Page Cellular uses the Verizon network and offers pre-paid plans ranging from $29.95 to $39.95 per month. These phones do not require SIM cards. PagePlus phones start at $39.95. Other phones that work well with Page Plus are Verizon contract phones, Android 1,2,3; HTC Incredible 1,2; and Droid X 1,2.

Utilities companies which provide gas & electric typically have programs for individuals/families going through economic medical hardship. Savings range from 20-35%. Some companies will make the switch over the phone while others will require you to fill out a form.

Other Bills

Besides these bills, ask your other monthly providers like child care, landlord, YMCA, etc. if they would give you a discount while you are going through cancer treatment. Don't be wishy-washy about it and be proactive. Make sure you emphasize that you are being up front and honest about your medical situation.

I have helped people get $300 reduction on their rent for a three month period and I personally reduced childcare by 25%. Property Taxes can be paid on an extended period if you ask although counties tend not to reduce the amount.

How To Reduce The Fat From Your Grocery Bills

Groceries are another expense that can be reduced immediately without giving up quality.

Health Food Stores are a great place to find nutritionally dense foods and often at great prices. I love the bins which all health food stores have. They usually have nuts, dried fruit, cereals, powdered soups, granola, pretzels, and crackers. You can buy as little or as much as you want, spending from 25 cents to 25 dollars per item.

Health Food Stores also have a fantastic fruit and vegetable selection. Buy what's in season because those items will be the best tasting with the lowest prices.

Visit www.organicconsumers.org to find a list of health food stores across the country.

I will have a booklet coming out in the next few months to show people how to set up a low cost healing kitchen so you can make simple and quick meals that will benefit your health & healing when you have cancer.

Grocery Chains obviously also carry fruits and vegetables, fish, meat etc. Buy what's in season as discussed above. The food will taste better and it will be less expensive. Grocery stores also have products on sale all the time. You'll find these items on the perimeter of the store.

99 Cents Store www.99only.com carries all types of food and produce all for that's right 99 Cents. Sometimes they carry organic fruits and vegetables as well. They have 256 locations across California, Arizona, Nevada and Texas.

Trader Joe's www.traderjoes.com is a great place to get low cost hormone and pesticide free eggs, milk and juices. They also have an amazing selection of prepared foods which will make your life easier when you don't feel up to cooking. As of the summer of 2013, TJ's has 437 locations nationwide.

Where To Find Free And Low Cost Delivered Meals

Jewish Family Services is a social service agency with locations in major cities throughout the US. Each location has a food bank where anyone in need can go for dry staples like cereal, tuna fish, canned soups, cookies, etc. The food bank is available to all people in need in the community. Also of note: there are no lines like other food banks.

It's the most dignified food bank in the country. To find the Jewish Family Services near you google JFS + your city -For example JFS San Diego or JFS New York.

Meals on Wheels www.mowaa.org **tel: 888-998-6325**

MOW can deliver one hot meal per day Monday - Friday and two cold meals for the weekends if requested. MOW's asks for a suggested price per meal of $4.00 and $3.00 per meal on the weekends but meals will be delivered whether you pay the full amount, partial or can't afford to pay at all.

Available in most areas of the country. When you visit their website it looks as if they only assist seniors but they also provide help to people who are disabled. Some local MOW's offer grocery shopping service.

In God's Love We Deliver www.glwd.org **212-294-8102**

God's Love We Deliver is the New York Tri-State area's leading provider of nutritious, individually-tailored meals to people who are too sick to shop or cook for themselves.

Founded in 1985 when one woman began delivering food on her bicycle to a man dying from AIDS, God's Love now cooks 4,600 meals each weekday, delivering them to clients living with life-altering illnesses in all five boroughs of New York City, Newark and Hudson County, New Jersey. All of their services are provided free of charge to their clients, their children and to the senior caregivers of our senior clients, without regard to income, and they have no waiting list. They deliver food within 24 - 48 hours of first being contacted.

How To Find Free Short, Medium, And Long Distance Transportation

Local Volunteer Driving Assistance

Road To Recovery www.cancer.org **800-227-2345**

Every day thousands of cancer patients need a ride to treatment, but some may not have a way to get there.

The American Cancer Society Road to Recovery program provides transportation to and from treatment for people who have cancer who do not have a ride or are unable to drive themselves. Volunteer drivers donate their time and the use of their cars so that patients can receive the life-saving treatments they need.

Bus & Train Assistance for Distances of 70-250 Miles One Way

The Angel Bus 800-768-0238   info@angelbus.org   is a nonprofit organization   providing   non-emergency   long distance   ground transportation to patients in need free of charge. A typical trip is 70-250 miles one way. **Amtrak, Greyhound and Trailways** participate in this program.

Long Distance Travel Flight Assistance

The National Patient Travel Center provides information about all forms of charitable, long-distance medical transportation and provides referrals to all appropriate sources of help available in the national charitable medical transportation network.

The purpose of the National Patient Travel Center is to ensure that no patient is denied access to distant specialized medical evaluation, diagnosis or treatment for lack of a means of long-distance medical transportation.

The National Patient Travel Center

www.patienttravel.org

800-296-1217

National Patient Travel Center has many resources at its disposal to assist patients.

National Patient Travel HELPLINE More than 14,000 calls were received by this HELPLINE last year. After an initial screening of patient need and determination of a suitable means of travel, callers are referred to the most appropriate charitable medical transportation program that can best meet their needs. This is a referral service and there is no cost for the information. This HELPLINE is available 24/7. A growing list of national medical and disease organizations utilize this HELPLINE to assist t h e i r constituency with charitable medical transportation information and referral.

How To Find Free And Low Cost Complementary Medicine

Acupuncture

Many people who have cancer would love to have acupuncture but the high cost per session will prevent them from going. Sessions with an acupuncturist can run from $65 to $350 per session depending on where you live and what the market will bear.

If you want to try acupuncture, but the cost is prohibitive, here are some suggestions:

Call your insurer and ask whether your policy covers acupuncture. Find out how many sessions a year it allows and whether a doctors prescription is needed. Check whether it allows coverage for cancer, pain, stress, nausea. Some policies, for instance, might cover acupuncture only for chronic pain.

Find an Accredited Acupuncture School in your area at www.acaom.org

The training lasts for 3 to 4 years depending on the state and the degree. I have been to schools throughout California and usually pay $15-$20. Explain your medical condition to them and ask for one of the more experienced students. Also you will benefit from having one of the professors present.

Community Acupuncture Centers can be found at www.pocacoop.com

Fees can be as low as $15 a session. You will receive a brief assessment and then are treated, fully clothed, in an open room with other patients. It is the acupuncture equivalent of a chair massage. Again, make sure that you ask for the most experienced Acupuncturist with experience dealing with cancer patients.

Pranic Healing www.pranichealing.com

Pranic Healing is a highly evolved and tested system of energy medicine developed by GrandMaster Choa Kok Sui that utilizes prana to balance, harmonize and transform the body's energy processes. Prana is a Sanskrit word that means life-force.

This invisible bio-energy or vital energy keeps the body alive and maintains a state of good health. In acupuncture, the Chinese refer to this subtle energy as Chi. It is also called Ruach or the Breath of Life in Hebrew.

There are free clinics all over the world for this type of healing. I used it to reduce stress during my treatments and for about a year after. It was a huge gift. It looks like hocus pocus but it works! It reduced my stress down to nothing. I felt like a Buddhist monk after these treatments! I became so relaxed in fact that I needed to sit down before driving.

Each center has a tip jar. Please be as generous as possible. These people offer this incredible service for free to their communities.

Biofeedback www.biofeedback.com

Biofeedback is another amazing tool for reducing stress, giving you another opportunity to improve your health. The problem is it's very expensive. Each session can easily cost $150-$250. The website listed above lists low cost options for portable and easy to use biofeedback.

Where To Find Free And Lower Cost Genetic Testing

Many of us followed news of Angelina Jolie recent decision to have a double mastectomy in May of 2013. In addition, she is also planning to have her ovaries removed, after learning that she carried a gene mutation linked to breast and ovarian cancers.

Jolie carries a mutation in a gene called BRCA1. According to the American Cancer Society, defects in that gene and another, called BRCA2, substantially raise a woman's lifetime risks of breast and ovarian cancers -- to a roughly 60 percent chance of developing breast cancer, and a 15 to 40 percent risk of ovarian cancer.

Genetic Testing can give you information about your genetic predisposition towards a particular cancer. It can also give you, your genetic counselor and oncologist information to choose the most effective treatments for your type of Cancer. Please speak to your oncologist and genetic counselor to see if genetic testing could be useful in your specific situation.

Myriad Genetics, Inc. offers an array of genetic tests, prognostic tests and personalized medicine tests to help healthcare providers assess a patient's increased cancer risk, disease aggressiveness and optimize efficacy of chemotherapy. Myriad's testing products can provide healthcare providers with information to help make medical management decisions to reduce cancer risk and help make sure specific treatments are tailored for each individual patient.

Beginning July 22, 2013, Myriad began offering financial assistance to qualified underinsured patients out-of-pocket cost to no more than $375. To be eligible, patients must have private insurance, meet their insurance's coverage criteria for testing, and meet low income requirements (household incomes up to 200 percent of the Federal poverty level). This expansion of Myriad's financial assistance program to underinsured patients complements the free testing Myriad currently offers for low income uninsured patients.

Myriad offers testing at no charge to uninsured patients that meet specific financial and medical criteria. Patients with insurance that meet similar financial and medical criteria may be eligible for financial assistance through Myriad. Due to regulatory limitations, patients who are recipients of government funded programs (ie, Medicaid, Medicare) are not eligible to apply for MFAP.

Qualification requirements and the submission instructions are provided below:

Myriad Financial Assistance Application

https://www.myriadpro.com/financial-assistance-programs/

To view the current HHS financial guidelines, please view the link below.

http://aspe.hhs.gov/poverty/index.shtml

There was a Supreme Court ruling in June, 2013 stating that Myriad doesn't hold the patent on the Human Gene and therefore can't corner the market on genetic testing for BRCA Testing for Breast and Ovarian Cancers. Please read the article for more information. Myriad has several competitors who will shortly be coming out with more affordable BRCA Testing.

http://blogs.wsj.com/law/2013/07/12/myriad-genetics-presses-ahead-after-high-court-ruling-on-patents/

Here is the Directory from National Cancer Institute to locate the genetic counselor and testing information by location and type of cancer. I don't have financial assistance information at this point, but you should ask what options there are for financial assistance.

http://www.cancer.gov/cancertopics/genetics/directory

When I had breast cancer I wanted to be tested for the BRCA gene because I have a long family history of lung, pancreatic, and other cancers that I couldn't get specific information about. I couldn't afford the test so I made a presentation to the hospital board of twenty people at one of their luncheons. There was zero time for humility. I don't think any other patient had done this. The board agreed to pay for the most basic BCRA test which was $540. The more comprehensive tests cost between $3000 to $7000.

How To Get Your Home Cleaned For Free (For Women Only)

Cleaning for a Reason - www.cleaningforareason.org is a non-profit organization which partners with maid services in the United States and Canada to offer professional house cleaning for women undergoing treatment for all types of cancer. Each women with cancer is offered one general house cleaning per month for four consecutive months. Bear in mind that this service doesn't guarantee there will be a maid service available in your area when you apply, but this service will continue to look for maid services in your area.

How To Go On A Free Cruise If You Have Cancer Or Are Recovering

Kick Cancer Overboard

The mission of KCO is to give away free cruises to people whose lives have been affected by cancer. They organize one free cruise per year.

Contact KCO to learn more.

Kick Cancer Overboard
Dr. James Parker Blvd Suite 104 Red Bank, NJ 07701

(732) 758-1990
kickit@kickcanceroverboard.org

How To Get A Free Spa Certificate If You Are A Woman Who Has Cancer

Heaven's Door Cancer www.heavensdooropen.com

Heaven's Door provides free spa trips (Diva Aftercare) to women fighting cancer across the U.S., to build and maintain self-esteem. This is a wellness spa treatment and advocacy program for women with cancer and advanced life threatening illnesses. Heavens Door purpose is Diva Aftercare Daphne Evans, the founder, is a multi-cancer survivor: ovarian, breast and spinal cancer.

Free spa visits or spa gift certificates are offered nationwide and recipients are seen by trained and licensed oncology and massage therapists.

CRITERIA:

In the middle of your battle; by recent surgery or recurrence of your cancer.

On chemo/radiation treatments.

Those who have recently come into remission up to 1 year.

Where To Order The Most Beautiful Silk Head Wraps For Free

Free Silk Headscarves

info@goodwishesscarves.org

888-778-5998

Good Wishes provides an It's a Wrap or Good Wishes square scarf to anyone experiencing the thinning or loss of hair as a result of illness or treatment at no cost. I wore one of these scarves every day after my hair fell out from the chemo. I didn't see any other women in the chemo room wearing interesting head scarves. These scarves are luxurious-beautiful, elegant, colorful, fun and otherwise purchased at Nordstrom's for $80!

Good Wishes will send you one free It's a Wrap or Good Wishes square scarf in the pattern and color of your choosing! To receive a complimentary wrap or scarf fill in the online request form or call. Someone from Good Wishes will respond within 48-72 hours. If you do not hear back please contact them or resubmit your request.

How To Get Free Gift Cards When You Have Cancer

The Cancer Card Exchange

info@cancercardexchange.org

The Cancer Card Exchange is a non profit organization that collects monetary and gift card donations and then distributes them to verified cancer patients.

According to the Tower Group Research Firm, $41 billion dollars worth of money on gift cards has gone unclaimed.

Please continue to look for other Health Correspondent booklets by Julie L. Kaye coming out soon. If you have questions or comments I would love to hear from you. I work as a health consultant and speaker and will tailor a program according to your needs.

You can contact me at julielkaye@gmail.com

Acknowledgements

There are many people to thank including my dear friend from Columbia University, Laura Betye who has a rare combination of intuition, intelligence and Romanian Gypsy in her. She told me not long ago that my astrological chart had publishing and writing all over it, and I told her she was crazy!

I would not be here today if it wasn't for both the administration at Scripps Hospital and The National Breast and Cervical Cancer Early Detection Program. It's hard to think of words to describe my gratitude.

I would like to thank Dr. Neysa Whiteman , my gynecologist at the time, for referring me to Dr. Mark Sherman. I am forever grateful to Dr. Sherman, aka Dr. Handsome, my surgeon, who read my mammograms, ultrasounds and biopsy reports for three years in a row and told me after the surgery, that it took him seventeen years of experience to be capable of that intricate a mastectomy. Any patient fortunate enough to have Dr. Sherman is in the best hands.

In addition, I would like to thank Pam and Vicki, the nurses at Pacific Oncology & Hematology Associates at Scripps Hospital who always offered their ear and warmth. Although it took awhile to be become entrenched in their system I wound up with two extraordinary medical social workers from JewishFamily Services, Gianna Muir-Robinson and later Stacie Saenz.

Lastly, the following people went out of their way on multiple occasions to help Eleanor and me; Lisa Nelson, Vivian Soderholm-Difatte, Brian Martin, Eva Meier, Sharon Wampler, Bart Ziegler, the staff from Montessori School of Encinitas, Breast Cancer Solutions, Marcia Donziger, the lovely Gina from Dr. Sherman's office and all thirty- nine families from Group 6 who went to China with us to adopt our beloved children..